ISBN-9
Library of Congress 2007906747
Second Edition

Guide to Caregiving in the Final Months of Life

This booklet is published by

TM Brown Publishers
21200 Hibbs Bridge Road
Middleburg, Virginia 20117

Voice Mail: 571-213-3845
FAX: 540-687-6212

Bulk Discounts are Available

To order go to our web site
www.GuidetoCaregiving.com
Or
See last page of this book for quick order form
Email: BetsyMurphyCHPN@aol.com

Cover photo by Stephen Blair
Cover Design by Julie Fanning Designs

Table of Contents

ABOUT THE AUTHOR

Betsy Murphy, FNP, CHPN, has worked in hospice care for 23 years in the Washington metropolitan area. Trained as a family nurse practitioner and certified as a hospice and palliative care nurse, she found the field of hospice work of great interest and has devoted her career to improving end-of-life care for patients and their families.

In recent years, Betsy's focus has shifted from hands-on nursing to that of an educator's role, teaching nurses, social workers, and the general public how to effectively work with patients in their final stages of life. In her own experience, she has found that both patients and families gained from caregiving experiences, and felt more in control of their individual situations, when an early identification was made of end-of-life signs.

As a board member of the Alzheimer's Association of the National Capital Area from 1995 to 2003, Betsy's influence brought a better understanding, locally and nationally, to dealing with the barriers to hospice and pain management for an often under-served population.

Widely published in nursing journals and a frequent speaker on hospice care, Betsy also recently wrote a chapter on end of life care for a nursing textbook. She was prompted to write her own book after watching many caregivers struggle to understand how to serve as an advocate for a loved one in the acute care setting.

A resident of Middleburg, Virginia, Betsy was recognized in 1997 and 2003 as an Outstanding Woman of Loudoun County by the Loudoun County Board of Supervisors. In 1993, she was honored as an Outstanding Woman in Medicine also by the Loudoun County Board of Supervisors.

Acknowledgments

I want to thank my hospice colleagues who reviewed the material, Michelle Thrush LCSW, Barbara Watts CHPN, Dixie Orrison CHPN, Deb Harney RN, Leah Grubbs LCSW and Clare Higgins RN, HTP. Ron Culberson MSW,CSP. I want to also thank family members, Mary Hibbard RN, MS, Joe Murphy MD, Susan Murphy PMHMT and Annie Murphy Roberts LMT and hospice volunteer.

I want to also thank friends who shared their personal experiences and insights, Cathi George CRNP, Melissa Hess MA, Marilyn Finnemore PhD, Marilyn Jarvis, Jan Spink MA and Diane Younkins MS,LGPC,NCC. Special thanks to my editor, Linda Roberts of Linda Roberts Communication, LLC.

Most importantly, I want to thank the hundreds of patients and their families who have been my best teachers, openly sharing their own journeys with me so I may better understand and serve others.

Disclaimer

This book is designed to provide information to caregivers to assist in advocating for a loved one. It is intended to provide caregivers and decision makers with baseline medical information that will help them in discussing the care of a loved one with their providers. It is intended to help broach the important subjects of goals for care giving and comfort care.

Because care of a patient at end of life should be individualized, this book could not possibly address all the potential events and issues that may occur for every patient. For that reason, the material is intended to be a guideline only, and not as an ultimate resource. The purpose of this book is to educate. Therefore neither the author, the publishing company, or those involved with the book's publication shall have liability or responsibility to any person with respect to any loss or damage caused directly or indirectly by the information contained in this book.

The bitterest tears shed over graves are for words left unsaid and deeds left undone.

Harriet Beecher Stowe

Preface
It's About Time

Only 10% of Americans will die suddenly. [1] The rest of us (90 percent) will gradually deteriorate, losing weight and growing weaker and becoming more dependent on others for care, as we age or fall prey to a debilitating illness.

Perhaps because this process is so gradual, families and friends don't recognize the signs and consequently fail to adequately prepare. We don't have the vital conversations that reveal how and where our loved one wants to spend their final weeks...how they want their possessions disbursed..how they want to be remembered. We don't have the conversations that allow old misunderstandings to be voiced and forgiven ...memories and history to be shared...and true connection to be achieved.

I am hopeful that this book will support you on this intimate journey with your loved one. That it will serve as a road map to understanding life's final chapter. That it will help you hope for the best but prepare for the inevitable. And most importantly, when your loved one dies, I hope that it helps in achieving the deep comfort that comes from knowing that you did your very best in a difficult time.

Recognition and acceptance of the slow decline of health over a lengthy time period is difficult. In fact, many people who are declining still view themselves as managing just fine.

When my mother-in-law was leaving the nursing home to come back to her home, she had declined so much that we were discussing the need for in- home caregivers. She could barely walk, yet she could not understand that she needed help and resisted hiring someone. She insisted, "I am just not that sick." She died less than 48 hours later. Somehow, she just could not acknowledge her decline either to herself or her family

Family members also may want to deny how seriously ill their loved one is. It's only when we think back over several months that we can see the subtle signs of decline. Denial can be a way of protecting ourselves from the painful reality that we may soon lose our parent or loved one. But this same denial that is so helpful to us in being able to cope, also interferes with making the necessary plans to living life's final weeks as we want them to be.

In addition to denial on the part of both the patient and their loved ones, our culture does not recognize that death is the natural end to life. In our society's popular entertainment outlets, death is often viewed as the enemy. The enemy that should be fought until the fight is won or lost. No one considers that the fight itself may intensify or prolong suffering. Death is rarely portrayed as a welcomed relief for someone who has been ill and suffering for a long time.

That being said, it is very normal for us to refuse to see death as a possibility when someone we love is seriously ill. We may fear that even thinking about their death is a form of betrayal. It is only natural that we would want to see our loved one as surviving, even when the situation is dire.

If we have not watched others die, we are inexperienced and sometimes cannot understand how close our loved one may be to dying. We expect to see dramatic changes, and we may miss the subtle changes like weight loss and weakness which are also key indicators of decline.

It is emotionally painful to think about someone dying. How will we manage without them? We feel frightened and lost in our grief. It feels like things are moving too fast, so we try to slow things down.

We avoid visiting them at the hospital or we avoid participating in making important health care decisions for them. This too is normal. Sometimes we try to slow things down because we need more time. We may feel guilty because we have not spent enough time with our loved one, or even if we have spent time, we have not said the things we wanted to say.

It is important to remember, that the best gift that you can give your loved one now is to take excellent care of *yourself.* The quality of your care giving and attentiveness for others is directly related to the care you take of yourself. Take breaks. Eat regularly. Talk to a friend about what is happening. Ask for help. Tell people what helps you and what doesn't.

Whatever you do, don't shut off the pain. Avoiding feelings will prolong your suffering. You will find that expressing your feelings will reduce your fatigue, clear your thoughts, and leave you stronger to care for the one you love.

—-Betsy Murphy FNP, CHPN

Chapter One
Life's Final Stage

Weight loss, increasing dependency, and inability to fight infections

For most elderly people, decline in the final years of life is so gradual that their loved ones may not notice. Families may be shocked when the nursing home tells them their loved one is losing weight or eating poorly. Weight loss alone may be the biggest indicator of decline in the elderly. There are many research studies which show that elderly people with 5-10 percent loss of body weight over a period of months have a very good chance of dying in the next six months even when they do not have a chronic disease.[2] [3] [4] We want to believe that feeding them more or using different kinds of food will help with weight gain and strength.

We may find ourselves becoming angry and wanting to blame caregiving staff for allowing them to lose weight. However, elderly people approaching the final months of life naturally stop wanting food and fluids. And for them, additional food will not extend life. In fact, forcing them to eat may create additional suffering. The section, "No Appetite" in Chapter Two explains why.

Weight loss by itself will cause loss of muscle, making the patient weaker and more dependent on others for care. As health further deteriorates, the immune system will be compromised and the body becomes vulnerable to infections. Two sites that tend to develop infections are the urinary tract and lungs.

Pneumonia

Before the widespread use of antibiotics in the 1940s, many elderly people died of pneumonia. So many people, that pneumonia was once called, "the old man's friend," as it promised a swift death.

We may think of pneumonia as being *curable*, but many elderly people continue to die from pneumonia, or its complications. If a person is older than 75 years, their chance of getting pneumonia is six times greater than if they were less than 60 years old.[5] [6] Once the person develops pneumonia, their ability to survive depends on their degree of health prior to getting sick. For example, many studies have shown that patients, who were in a wheelchair or bedridden at the time of contracting pneumonia, were less likely to survive the pneumonia.[7] [8] People who are recently confused and those with dementia also have a greater chance of dying from pneumonia.[9] [10]

A final and important point is that after the first time an elderly person develops pneumonia, *even if they recover*, the chance of their dying in the next one to four years is now greatly increased. [11] [12] [13]

So the elderly person who is bed-and-chair bound and confused is likely to die from pneumonia or to die soon after the episode of pneumonia. For many elderly who are weak and confused an episode of pneumonia may be an indication that they are in the final months of life. In fact, pneumonia is a leading cause of hospitalization and death for nursing home residents. [14]

Below are some examples in question and answer format to assist in understanding *Life's Final Stages.*

Example

My 92-year-old father has been gradually losing weight and getting weaker since last year. He is now bed bound and has been sent to the hospital by the nursing home because they suspect he has a urinary tract infection. What can be done to help him?

With your father's history of gradual decline, it's very possible that he is in the final months of life. The hospital will find and treat his infection, but since he has been declining for a year it's likely that he will continue to decline after his infection is treated. [15] This is a good time to meet with his providers to discuss future care goals. During this hospital stay, you can ask to talk with a hospice representative about hospice care. He or she will be able to tell you if your father's condition is appropriate for hospice care or when he will be appropriate. With hospice in place in the nursing home, they can assure his final months are comfortable and provide you with information about treatment options to promote comfort.

Example

My mother has been ill with dementia for more than 10 years. She lives in a nursing home and has been unable to get out of bed for several months. The nursing home has sent her to the hospital to be treated for pneumonia. Now she is unconscious and is in intensive care. I am her designated medical decision maker and I am wondering if we are adding to her suffering.

Because she has advanced dementia, increasing dependency, and is no longer conscious, she is at high risk for dying from her pneumonia. As her decision maker, you are right to be evaluating the benefits and burdens of her treatment. You also have a legal right as her decision maker to refuse any medical treatment that you believe may not be benefiting her.

It may be helpful to start by defining goals for her care. If your goal is to maximize comfort, then you can tell her providers that comfort is what is most important to you now. Then, the focus of her care can be directed to managing symptoms and assuring comfort.

Sepsis

Sepsis is a condition where an infection, like pneumonia, has spread to the blood stream. Sepsis is a serious illness and the tenth most common cause of death in the United States.[16] Sometimes sepsis can become so severe that all the body systems respond. Through a series of complicated events, body temperature may increase or decrease. The heart beats faster, breathing is rapid and labored, and blood pressure drops making it difficult to get oxygen to essential body organs and tissues. The end result is organ damage or failure.

The body will attempt to preserve blood supply to the heart and brain by diverting blood from the kidneys, so the kidneys are commonly injured first. The intestines may be damaged and normal bacteria that live there may be absorbed into the blood stream causing infection. Liver injury can occur causing problems with bleeding. The immune system itself is affected, depleting the body's defenses, and leaving it more vulnerable to infection. This is all happening at a time when the body needs more oxygen to function. When interventions fail to improve sepsis, it will lead to septic shock, a life threatening condition.

Because there is inadequate delivery of oxygen and nutrients to body tissues, the end result is organ failure or damage.

Sepsis is the leading cause of death in intensive care units. [17] Mortality is high, somewhere between 28 and 80 percent. Most likely to die from sepsis are the elderly, due to organ failure and multiple medical conditions. Some will survive the sepsis while hospitalized. However, those same survivors will continue to have an increased chance of dying, because of sepsis for the next five years. [17]

And for many, their quality of life will be reduced because of the aftermath of sepsis. They will continue to suffer with depression, weakness, shortness of breath and fatigue. Many of these elderly will realize their worst fears and will be unable to return to their own homes and will go to nursing facilities.

In summary, the process of aging even without a disease creates problems with weight loss progressive weakness and difficulty fighting infections. This will directly affect the elderly person's ability to survive when they have a medical crisis.

Compounding this problem, we often send frail elderly people to the hospital when they have an infection. Studies show that elderly people lose ground while in the hospital. [18] [19] Some will lose weight and others will return home weaker than before they went to the hospital. Being confined to the hospital, by itself, will cause an elderly person to decline.

In addition, all elderly people who are moved from familiar surroundings will inevitably suffer some loss as a result of the move. They will go through a period of sadness as they grieve this loss and adjust to their new surroundings. Changes in living situations however, often become necessary. The key is to be sure that if your loved one needs to move, make sure that they can remain in their new environment for the remainder of their days.

On the following page are some more *examples* in question and answer format to assist in understanding "Life's Final Stages."

Examples

My frail 94-year-old aunt came to the hospital with a urinary infection, and now she is confused and in intensive care. We were told that she has sepsis and that her kidneys are failing. Her providers are suggesting dialysis.

Because she was frail and elderly *before* coming to the hospital, she will have difficulty in fighting infections. She also is likely to continue to lose weight and grow weaker while in the hospital especially since she is now confused. Her frailty, age, and organ failure will make recovery very difficult.

My grandfather has been a nursing home resident for 15 years. He got an infection which turned into sepsis at the hospital and now he is returning to the nursing home, more confused and weaker. We don't want to put him through something like this again. What can we do?

You can talk with your health care provider and the nursing home about having a *Do Not Hospitalize* order on his chart. That means when he becomes ill again, he can be treated at the nursing home and will not be sent to the hospital. Keeping him in his familiar environment with his familiar caregivers will reduce his stress. You can ask for your local hospice to assess him for hospice care. The hospice team will provide you with treatment options as his condition changes in the facility. The booklet, *Hard Choices for Loving People* by Hank Dunn (A&A Publishers) will be very helpful to you now in making decisions.

My elderly grandmother was brought to the hospital after she fell at home. She has been losing weight for the last year and getting weaker and is more confused. The hospital staff is insisting that they must feed her artificially to see if she will get stronger. But she has always told us she did not want a feeding tube. What should we do? Who can help us with this?

A hospital ethics committee can be very helpful in cases like your grandmother's where there is disagreement between you and the providers about her care. A patient or a family member can contact the hospital ethics committee and request a consultation.

The role of the ethics consultant is to provide education on ethical issues. The ethics committee is knowledgeable about legal and ethical issues, including patients rights. A representative will review her medical record, help sort through the important issues, and improve the communication between you and your grandmother's health care providers to help you to arrive at the best possible decision. They will not tell you what they think you should do but they will help you to arrive at the decision that best reflects her wishes and values.

The next chapter describes how an elderly person's body is less efficient than a younger person, and why the same treatments that are effective for the young may fail to heal and may even hurt the elderly.

We don't see things as they are.
We see things as we are.

Talmud

Chapter Two
Why Recovery is Not Possible

No Appetite

Elderly people in the final months of life have reduced appetites. They may not feel hungry and when they are hungry, they tend to eat less. As we age, our sense of smell and taste are reduced. For those taking medications, the taste of food may be altered and unpleasant because of the medications. Many elderly people don't feel thirsty, so they do not drink enough fluids.This makes their mouth feel dry which in turn makes swallowing difficult. Chewing may also be difficult due to poor dental health, loss of teeth, or ill-fitting dentures. Everything about the body is slowing down. As the stomach empties slowly, the person may feel full, sometimes even after just a few bites of food. The tendency is to eat small amounts during the day instead of the larger meals that they ate in the past. These changes in diet and activity can lead to constipation, which contributes to their already poor appetite and can make them feel ill. Thus begins a cycle of eating less, which causes increased weakness. Weakness causes loss of muscle. Loss of muscle, in turn, causes even more weakness.

Progressive Weakness

Progressive weakness is another sign that someone may be approaching the final months of life. This may start with a person's inability to get out of the chair without help. It will naturally progress to needing assistance to get out of bed and maybe even needing the help of two people to move from bed to chair. This decrease in activity goes hand in hand with weight loss and loss of muscle. Often there is nothing you can do that will make them stronger. Some families will ask for physical therapy to help get their loved one stronger. A consult with a physical therapist may give you information as to whether the weakness is reversible or not. In the final months and weeks of life, all patients will move around less and the focus of their care will shift from protecting them when they are walking to caring for them while they are confined to the bed and or chair.

At Risk for Pneumonia

Just as the stomach and digestion is affected by the aging process, so too are the lungs, which are less flexible and do not expand and contract easily. Limited expansion means they take in less oxygen. You will notice that the patient gets short of breath with even slight exercise.

Remember earlier when we said that oxygen is essential for *all* body processes? This change in the ability to take in and use oxygen can make the person feel tired and act confused. Making it worse, breathing becomes shallow and they not only take in less air but they also are not able to completely empty the lungs when air is exhaled. As a result, carbon dioxide builds up in the lungs. This buildup can cause yet more difficulty breathing.

One of the most dangerous changes in the aging lung is that an elderly person is no longer able to effectively cough up mucus. Changes in the brain and nervous system affects the elderly person's ability to swallow; they may choke, accidentally inhaling liquid into the lungs. They may even choke on their own saliva, inhaling it into their lungs. This is called aspiration. This accidentally inhaled liquid is a problem, as it includes bacteria from the mouth, which can cause an infection in the lungs.

Aspiration itself is not a problem with young, healthy people. Young people may aspirate while choking or even while sleeping but they are able to effectively cough up mucous and their healthy immune systems can effectively fight the infection.

Elderly people, on the other hand, are unable to cough effectively causing the liquid to remain in the lungs. Because this problem with aspiration is often not reversible, it means that they will have repeated episodes of pneumonia. The pneumonia may be successfully treated the first time, but each episode will further weaken the body, making recovery less likely. This condition also affects the person's ability to eat; they will lose more weight, become drowsy, and they may have side effects from the antibiotics themselves.

Heart Trouble and Organ Failure

As we age, we also experience age-related changes in heart and blood vessels. With this wear and tear from aging, some people will go on to develop disease of the heart or blood vessels. Heart disease accounts for half the deaths in people over 65 years old. Your loved one may or may not have been diagnosed with a heart condition, but age, nevertheless, is changing their heart and blood vessels.

Blood vessels, which carry necessary oxygen, become narrower and less flexible, making it harder for the oxygen to get to the brain, liver and kidneys. Secondly, the heart pump is weaker and the heart beat may be less regular. A weak pump combined with smaller blood vessels adds up to less oxygen traveling to the organs.

Without oxygen, organs will start to fail. If the heart beat is irregular, the heart itself is deprived of oxygen, which will damage the heart. These changes make a person vulnerable to many things. Problems with fluid congestion may develop. You may notice this in the form of swelling in the legs, but there is also fluid congestion in places you cannot see, such as the lungs and liver. Congestion in the lungs makes it even harder to take in oxygen, and less oxygen in the lungs means less life-giving oxygen transported to the kidneys and liver. Damage to the liver and kidneys reduces the body's ability to remove medications from the body. Medications can reach toxic levels and these toxic levels can cause more organ damage.

The failure of one organ will lead to the failure of another.

The organs of the body are dependent on one another to do their jobs properly. As you will see from the example above, when one organ is having difficulty, it will affect another organ's ability to do its job properly, or it may even damage that organ. As the kidneys malfunction, they will not be able to process the medications, which will result in toxic levels of the medication in the body. Toxic levels can result in nausea, confusion and more weakness. At some point, it may be difficult to tell if medicines are helping or making the situation worse. For that reason, many medications are stopped in the final days of life except for comfort medications.

Because the person is fragile, each setback makes recovery less likely. Family members who find their loved one in intensive care are often confused by this and wonder why organs can't be repaired. Making their confusion worse is that each organ may be managed by a specialist, who will fight hard to improve that organ's function. It may be difficult to have an overview of the patient and his or her chance of survival. Without that, decision making will be challenging. It is clear, however, that once elderly people have failure of multiple organs, they have a very poor chance of survival.

Fighting Infections

It is commonly known that there is a progressive decline in the power of the immune system with aging. As stated earlier, this is related to changes in nutrition and insufficient oxygen. Also, elderly patients will not show the same signs of infection that younger people do. They often don't run a fever and may not cough. Instead, they will be confused or weak. So their infection may be diagnosed and treated later, and this also affects their ability to recover. Antibiotics will be less effective because the body is less effective in fighting the infection. Elderly people with pneumonia, who find themselves in intensive care units, will have very poor survival rates. 20

Example

My wife is 87, with dementia, and has been losing weight for a year. She is having trouble swallowing and the hospital tells me that she is inhaling fluid into her lungs when she eats. Because she has had pneumonia once already, they are suggesting we put in a feeding tube. When she was well, she never wanted a tube. What should I do?

Your local Alzheimer's association is a good resource for you (www.alz.org). They have a 24 hour Helpline ;the number is 800-272-3900. Tube feeding is no longer encouraged for people with end stage dementia as research has shown that they do not gain weight or live longer. 21 Using proper hand-feeding techniques is the solution. Ask for a palliative care or hospice consultation.

Example

My elderly mother is seriously ill and in intensive care. Each day we are told that some of her blood tests are better, but her heart and her kidneys are failing. Her body looks swollen and she does not recognize us anymore. What should we do?

You can ask for a meeting with her specialists to try and obtain a picture of her overall health. The more organs that are failing, the less likely that she will recover. Sometimes having a meeting with a palliative care specialist, or a hospice nurse can be helpful. The health care team in intensive care sometimes assumes that all patients want aggressive treatment. Some aggressive treatments can be uncomfortable. You can tell them that making sure that she is comfortable is very important to you now.

Chapter Three
At The End

Symptom: Fatigue and Weakness

As mentioned earlier, progressive weakness will begin to occur months before death. Your loved one will have good days and bad days. Days of lots of activity followed by days of mostly resting. In the final weeks, weakness will escalate and in the final hours the patient may be sleeping more than 16 hours a day. Sometimes they sleep during the day and are awake at night. This will be very difficult for caregivers, who are trying to provide care both day and night.

There are two important things to remember as the person grows weaker, keep them safe and protect their skin. Keeping them safe may be a challenge as the person often doesn't see themselves as weaker. Placing necessities near the bed or chair, encouraging use of a walker, and walking or standing next to them when they do activities may be helpful. Patients will sometimes test their physical limits and have a fall. This commonly happens no matter how hard you try to make them safe. Many patients will fall before they finally realize how weak they truly are. If your loved one does fall, remember that it is not your fault. It happens often when people grow weaker.

Lying in bed for long periods of time can be uncomfortable. To make the person more comfortable, they will need assistance to be turned and repositioned. A "draw" sheet, folded in half and placed under the trunk of the body, will make it easy to turn the person from side to side and to pull them up in bed. In the final hours of life, the person may no longer need turning as the motion may increase distress rather than promote comfort.

Also, in the final hours the person's eyes may appear unfocused and they may be unable to see. Hearing will continue until the end. They will also still feel your touch, best felt in the area around their heart.

In the final hours, they may not respond to you when you speak to them. It is natural that you would try and speak louder but that will not work. They do not respond because they are simply too weak to speak or to move. If there are things that you wanted to say but did not earlier, this would be a good time to do that. They will still be able to hear you.

Caregiving Tips: *If your loved one is awake at night and asleep during the day, it will be important for you to get adequate rest. Sometimes your health care provider can adjust or add medications to help them sleep at night. If this is not successful, hiring a night time caregiver will assure that the patient is safe and that you will get adequate rest to continue care giving during the day.*

A hospital bed will be very helpful for both patient and caregiver. The patient will be able to have more control, elevating head or feet, and the side rails will enable them to pull themselves up. Caregivers will be able to regulate the height of the bed to make turning them from side to side and caring for their skin easier. Keep the skin dry and warm.

Make a draw sheet by folding a sheet in half and placing it under the trunk of their body. With one person on each side of the bed, grasp the draw sheet at the top and the bottom and on the count of three, pull the patient up in the bed, and reposition them on their alternate side. Check their skin, especially at the base of the spine, the heels and elbows, and massage any pink areas with lotion.

Explain to them what you are doing. Touch can be comforting and again, they will feel your touch best near their heart.

Symptom:
Changes in Breathing Patterns

One of the most difficult changes for families is when they see a change in the way their loved one is breathing. Rapid breathing is distressing and families fear their loved one will suffocate. The good news is that breathing difficulties can often be easily managed. If breathing is rapid (more than 24 breaths per minute) and the person is working hard to breathe, morphine may be started.

Morphine is regarded as a medication for pain, but it is very helpful when someone has trouble breathing. With rapid breathing, each breath is shallow and less oxygen is taken in. Morphine will slow breathing so the person can take in more oxygen with each breath. Morphine also works on the part of the brain that feels short of breath to eliminate the perception of breathlessness. Sometimes the breathing may be accompanied by a rattling sound. This is caused by saliva collecting at the back of the throat since the person is unable to swallow it. Morphine will help dry up the saliva and reduce the sound. Some people worry that morphine will shorten their loved one's life. The experience of hospice staff has been that a gradual increase in morphine is safe and will not shorten the time they have left. 22

Caregiving Tips: *If someone is short of breath, morphine will need to be given regularly. You can tell when they are short of breath by counting their respirations.* ***If their respirations are more than 24-26 per minute and if they are using their muscles in their neck and stomach to breathe, you should seek help from their provider right away.***

Once morphine is started, you will need to give it regularly because if it is stopped, rapid breathing and throat secretions will come back. Morphine is usually given via dropper under the tongue. It will start to work in 10-20 minutes. You can count the number of respirations after 10 minutes to see if they are decreasing. Do not worry about giving 5 to 15 mg. of morphine every two to six hours. This low dose is well tolerated. Sometimes you can elevate the head of the bed, using gravity to help the secretions go down. Also positioning the person on their side may help. Some patients will benefit from oxygen. If you don't have oxygen, often just putting a fan on low speed, aimed at their nose and mouth will help reduce their sensation of breathlessness. Sometimes a moist humidifier in their room can help loosen secretions and make it easier for them to cough. There are additional medications available to help dry secretions if the morphine is not effective.

Symptom:
Stopping Eating and Drinking

In the final days and hours of life, the person is just not hungry. Swallowing and digesting food takes energy and their energy is depleted. At some point, they may clamp their mouth shut and refuse food. They may continue to take sips of fluids, but eventually they will also refuse fluids. Families worry that not eating or drinking will make them uncomfortable. Most experts feel that in the final hours of life, dehydration is not uncomfortable and may in fact stimulate the release of endorphins in the body to promote comfort. [23 24] So most dying patients will not require artificial fluids. There are, however, some patients who may benefit from receiving intravenous (IV) fluids.

An example is the patient who requires constant blood levels of a drug. Patients with severe pain or severe shortness of breath will require continuous morphine or another opioid. Giving morphine continuously will assure that no doses are missed and comfort is constant. This is often done in a hospital setting. Another type of patient who may benefit from low volume artificial fluids is one having side effects from their body's inability to process a drug. The drug byproducts build up and they may develop agitation.

Caregiving Tips: *Offer small amounts of favorite foods regularly during the day. Soft foods like ice cream, custard, yogurt, and applesauce require less chewing and are easier to swallow. Avoid preparing foods with offensive odors as this will affect appetite. Moist foods will be easier to swallow than dry foods. Foods with sauces or gravies may be better tolerated. Expect that at some point, solid food will be refused because of difficulty in swallowing and fear of choking. Remind yourself that forcing them to eat will not make them live any longer. While feeding your loved one has been a source of joy and love, food is no longer something that they want or require. However, touch is something that is needed. Massaging lotion into their skin, foot massage, and just being with them will be appreciated.*

Their mouth may feel dry, so moisten it by using a straw dipped in water, placing the drops on their tongue. Toothette swabs can be dipped in water and swabbed in the mouth every 30 minutes to maintain moisture. Some patients will even actively suck water from the toothette. Lemon glycerin swabs should not be used as they will tend to be more drying over the long run. Coat the lips with a thin layer of petroleum jelly to prevent cracking. If using oxygen, a non-petroleum-based product in the nose will work best to make sure the oxygen tubing is not blocked. If needed, artificial tears in the eyes every three to four hours will prevent dryness.

Decisions about hydration should be made according to the needs of each patient. The majority of people dying at home will be very comfortable dehydrating naturally. Artificial hydration will not be necessary. Families and significant others can be relied upon to give medications regularly and to provide mouth care.

This can be a difficult time for families who have taken pride in the feeding of their loved one. Instead of feeding, finding new ways to communicate their caring such as gentle skin massage or regular mouth care is the key.

Symptom:
Managing Pain

Pain is under treated in this country. There are many reasons for this. Health care providers lack education about pain medication and fear government reprisal. Many patients who are in pain fear they will become addicted to medications. However, it's estimated that the rate of addiction for patients in pain is less than one percent. 25 Patients also erroneously believe that if they take the medication now, it will not work later when the pain is more severe. For these reasons you will see patients taking the least amount of medication needed to control pain.

Another problem in assessing pain is that pain perception varies from person to person and it's impossible to predict who will or won't have pain, or how much medication they will require for comfort.

When you care for your loved one, you may also find yourself becoming fearful of treating pain. Remember that there is also a price for inadequately treated pain. It has both physical and emotional consequences. Pain stresses the body, affecting its ability to fight infection. Because it hurts when they move, patients will not move and this reduced movement puts them at higher risk for blood clots and pneumonia. It compromises the heart and lung functioning.

Poorly controlled pain may actually hasten death. It creates poor quality of life, depression and despair. As stated earlier under the “Changes in Breathing Patterns” section, gradual increases of opioid medications for both pain and shortness of breath are safe and will not shorten life.

Below are some simple concepts about pain management that will help you in treating your loved one's pain.

Common Questions that Caregivers have about Treating Pain.

How can I tell if my loved one is in pain if they cannot tell me?

In the final days of life, many patients are unable to communicate that they are in pain. For that reason, if the patient has a condition with potential for causing pain, they should be treated for pain until it's proven that they are not in pain. Common signs of pain are: facial grimacing or frowning, irritability, refusing to move in bed, or crying out when moved or turned. Other signs are restlessness, confusion, pulling at tubes or dressings and persistent rubbing of parts of the body. People with Alzheimer’s or dementia will often show pain by resisting care, frowning or agitation.

My mother says she does not have pain but she is grimacing.

Most elderly people will deny having pain. They feel they should be able to endure a certain amount of pain. They also have several unspoken fears. They fear addiction, despite the fact that their chance of becoming addicted is less than one percent. 25 They fear that if they take the medications now, the drugs will lose power and not work later for them when the pain is worse. They may also fear becoming constipated.

The truth about pain is that experts feel that 95 percent of pain is controllable, even in the late stages of a disease. There is no limit to the amount of opioid medication they can take. If the opioid works today, it will continue to work, but they will require gradual increases in the dose as their body will become used to the drug.

In assessing pain, avoid using the word "pain" and try asking if they "hurt." Many older people think of "pain" as being severe. When you use the word "hurt" you are allowing them to acknowledge less severe pain. Have them define their "hurt" by a number. With zero being *no hurt* and 10 *the most hurt they can imagine*. Using numbers will give you a better idea of their level of pain.

Using numbers is also important

because you will have a way to measure if the medications are working or not. When you ask them their "pain number" one or two hours later, the number will go down if the medicine is working. Ask your health care provider to reassure them that they are not likely to become addicted. Have your provider also reassure them that pain can be controlled throughout their illness and that there is no limit to the amount of medications they can receive.

Constipation is a known side effect of pain medication. Make sure that they have been ordered medication to prevent constipation. Stool softeners and/or stimulants containing senna are very effective, but need to be taken daily in order to work.

My mother was in pain for several days and I started the pain medicine. Now she is sleeping all of the time.

For patients who are not actively dying, pain is exhausting. Often people in pain have slept poorly over a long period of time. Expect that they will catch up on their rest once the pain is well controlled. They should be less exhausted in 48 hours.

Some patients have increased pain because they are dying. The medication will not shorten their life, just make them more comfortable.

After I give the pain medication, how soon will it work and how long will the pain medicine last?

If you are giving a pill that is swallowed, it may take 30 minutes to an hour to see results. The medication will last two to six hours.

If you are giving medication by droplet under the tongue, it may take from 10 to 30 minutes to start working and will last two to six hours.

If you are giving an intravenous injection, the medication will start working in 10 minutes and may last one to three hours.

Rectal pain medications will usually work within 30 minutes.

When pain is severe or in the final days of life, it will be important to give the medication regularly. If you miss a dose and pain returns, it will take two consecutive doses to get the pain under control again. If they are in the final stages of their disease, remember that sleeping most of the day is expected in the final days of the dying process. The pain medication is not causing them to sleep, but it is assuring that they continue to be comfortable in those final hours.

What are the side effects of these medicines?

Initially, you can expect some sleepiness and sometimes nausea. Both of these should improve in time. Dry mouth is expected and needs to be managed from the beginning. Moist foods and ice chips will help the dry mouth.

Opioids will cause the bowel to slow down; making stools hard and difficult to expel. Constipation should be avoided by starting medications to prevent constipation with the first dose of the opioid. The goal is to have a bowel movement at least every three days. As stated above, stool softeners plus senna work well. A high fiber diet may not be effective because of insufficient fluid intake.

My father has advanced cancer and he is taking morphine for his pain. He wants to reduce the frequency of the medications and take it five times a day instead of six. He feels he should be able to endure some pain.

Pain medication for advanced cancer needs to be taken regularly. The short-acting medicines usually do not last longer than four hours. If a dose of pain medication is missed, then it will be eight hours between doses. The pain will usually come back and they will need two consecutive doses of the medication to bring the pain back under control. He will actually use less medication if he stays with his six doses a day regimen.

What if the pain medication I give causes my loved one to die?

There are two things to consider here. As discussed earlier, in the section on "Changes in breathing patterns," opioid medications when increased gradually and given regularly will not cause a premature death. In the final hours of life, the opioid medications are given regularly to keep blood levels of the medications constant. Because your loved one is dying and they cannot communicate, it's necessary to continue to give medications regularly to be sure that they stay pain free. It is expected that they will die at some point while receiving pain medication. This does not mean that the medication caused their death. Your intent is to relieve suffering and assure that they stay as comfortable as possible.

Are medicines the only way to control pain?

Some people may receive benefit from counseling, music therapy, meditation, etc. Some types of pain will improve with applying heat or cold or using massage.

Confusion

In the weeks and months before someone dies, there may be moments when your loved one provides information, in an unconventional way, that is helpful to family members. In the final days some patients will hallucinate and say that a deceased family member is in the room with them. They may say that their spouse is waiting for them. They may also talk about needing to catch a bus or a plane. They may ask about their passport. While it may seem as if they are living in two different worlds, this is often meaningful information for family members. To read more about the meaningful communication of the dying, read *Final Gifts*: *Understanding the Special Awareness, Needs, and Communications of the Dying,* (Random House) and written by Maggie Callanan and Patricia Kelley.

Often, patients who have been lethargic and confused for days will become awake and have some hours of complete mental alertness. This can be very confusing for caregivers. They may second guess themselves and their decisions and ask about resuming medical treatments. This gift of their presence is usually short-lived and most of them will continue to die within hours to days.

Caregiving tips: *Gently remind your loved one of the time, date, and people who are present. Be calm and reassuring. Keep a dim light on in the room. If they speak of others who have died, encourage them to talk about what is happening rather than correct them.*

Example

In the weeks before my father died, he was in the hospital with kidney failure caused by his heart failure.
He was giving instructions to me and my sister about his bay front property, which had flooded following Hurricane Isabel. He told us that during the hurricane he feared that he would drown. He also said that his septic system was now broken and we should not fix it. We later realized that he was not talking about his property, which had easily survived the hurricane, but rather about his body. That he fears drowning as a result of his heart failure, and that his kidneys were now "broken" and we were not to ask for dialysis.

Loss of Bowel or Bladder Control

Most patients will eventually lose control of their bladder. Sometimes they have control, but they lose the ability to tell you that they need to urinate. As they dehydrate naturally, their urine will become very dark in color and may have a strong odor. They may or may not lose control of the bowel.

Caregiving tips: *The simple solution is to use adult diapers and tell them to go ahead and urinate into the diapers. Catheters are usually not necessary, but can be helpful for some patients, keeping patients dry who have bedsores.*

Body Temperature Changes

The body will lose its ability to control temperature in the final days. The patient may be either very cold or may be hot and sweaty. You may notice that the fingertips or mouth are grey or blue. When the person's legs become mottled and blue, it's often an indication that they are in the final hours of life.

Caregiving tips: *Keep the patient as clean and dry as possible. Use blankets for warmth, but do not use heating pads or hot water bottles as there is a risk of burns. Change moist garments often.*

Terminal Restlessness

This is a syndrome seen in a number of patients in the final days of life. Some studies have shown that as many as 80 percent of dying patients will be restless. It may start as an inability to concentrate or relax. They may pick at the sheets with their fingers or at the air around them. They may just be mildly confused, but this confusion may escalate to hallucinations or trying to climb out of bed.

Caregiving tips: *It will be helpful to contact your health care provider* ***early*** *to obtain their help in determining the cause of the agitation. There are some causes that are reversible. If pain is the cause, it can be treated. If they have a full bladder and cannot urinate, a catheter can be inserted. If they are constipated, it can be managed. If the cause is side effects from medication, they may be stopped or reduced. A health care provider can often determine and reverse the cause. Because this situation can escalate and become less manageable, you will want to notify your home care on call service or your healthcare provider when you first notice changes. Early interventions will make a vast difference in the quality of your loved ones final hours and in your family's experience with the dying process.*

The Moment of Death

As stated earlier, usually the legs have become mottled and bluish. Normally the breathing will get erratic. They may have rapid breathing alternating with very slow breaths. The breaths will slow down and stop.

Signs that Death has Occurred

The heart stops beating
Breathing stops
Pupils become fixed and dilated
Skin becomes pale and waxen
Body temperature drops
Eyes remain open
Jaw drops open

Being Present at the Time of Death

Many family members want to be with their loved one at the moment of death. They keep a vigil almost twenty four hours per day. They leave the bedside only to get some food or to take a shower. Despite this, the patient sometimes dies the moment they leave the room. I have wondered if they do this intentionally to spare their wife, husband or children. We do not really know why. If this should happen to you, it is important for you to know that it happens quite often. Because you were not there at the moment of death in no way diminishes the quality of your loving care throughout their illness.

Love is the capacity to take care, to protect, to nourish. If you are not capable of generating that kind of energy toward yourself, of nourishing yourself, of protecting yourself-it is very difficult to take care of another person.

Thich Nhat Hanh

Chapter Four
Communication Considerations
Denial

Often patients who are in their final weeks of life talk about getting better. This hope for cure may seem unreasonable, but it may be necessary for them to talk about it in order to keep on living. Like my mother-in-law in the first chapter, most people cannot acknowledge the severity of their illness or the hopelessness of their recovery. They may do this to protect themselves or to protect their families. They may use their denial in order to function on a day-to-day basis. As we talked about in the introduction, denial can be a wall of protection to shield us from emotional pain. If we take away this wall, we can cause an unnecessary emotional crisis. Denial gives the dying person time to gather strength.

Allow your loved one to be where they are emotionally. Whether in denial or angry or sad, the day may come when they are ready to talk about it. Listen carefully in your daily conversations with them. And when they say, “I don’t think I will get better,” your instinct will be to say, “Of course you will,” but don’t say that. Instead say, “What will that mean for you?” In sharing their fears with you, they will feel less isolated and alone.

Just as your loved one is experiencing emotional ups and downs, you will find yourself vacillating between knowing your loved one will die and hoping that they will recover. This is normal.

Stressed caregivers, whose loved ones are in intensive care, may secretly wish for a quick and final resolution to the day-by-day emotional decision making. They also may find themselves overwhelmed with guilt after perhaps wishing that their loved one would die. This too is normal. People become mentally and physically exhausted after so many days of denying their own needs.

You may find yourself getting angry with your loved one for getting sick. You may get angry at yourself wondering if you had cared for him or her differently, would the illness have occurred? You may worry that you fed the wrong food, or wish that you had urged better care. All of these thoughts are normal.

When you find yourself struggling with these thoughts, it may be best to identify what it is you are feeling and say so.

I am angry with him (her) for not taking better care of himself (herself).

I am angry with myself for not insisting he (she) went to the doctor.

I am angry that my husband's (wife's) illness turned our world upside down.

It's important to be kind to yourself. Allow your feelings to exist as they are. Moods will come and go. Knowing what you are feeling can help release tension.

Anger

Many people become angry as a buffer to avoid anxiety and grief.

I remember the day the internist told my father that he had nothing more to use in treating his heart disease. My father walked out of the exam room to the full waiting room and turned and said with sarcasm, "Have a nice life."

Often anger is a result of fear. The dying person fears loss of control, being a burden to their family, becoming financially devastated. Above all, they fear suffering and that they will die alone. We can help them to talk about their anger, by asking questions “You seem very upset.” “Tell me what frightens you.” “So you are worried about running out of money?”

Anger is a normal part of grieving for the caregiver also. But in the hospital setting, if you are outwardly angry, health care providers may try to avoid you. Get help with your anger. The hospital social worker or chaplain would be a good source of support. Your anger is part of the process and it needs to be validated and expressed. Your anger is not a sign that you don’t love or care. It is more often a sign of fatigue and fear that you will be unable to manage the caregiving challenges ahead.

Sadness and emotional withdrawal are also a normal part of their grieving. Expect that your loved one will emotionally retreat in the final days of their life. Their physical and emotional energy is depleted and they are getting ready to go.

Some dying patients will feel that they cannot leave you. A husband may not want to leave behind a wife, feeling that he needs to continue to take care of her. It may be helpful in these situations to find a way to give them permission to go.

It may be helpful to say, “I love you, I will miss you and will never forget you. Do what you need to do when you are ready.”

Chapter Five
Hospice Care and Palliative Care

Some people think of hospice as being a place, but it is really a service. A service that brings care to you and your family. Hospice cares for people at home, but hospice care can also be provided in a number of different settings. It is available in a hospital or in a nursing home when the hospice has a formal contract with the facility. Hospice can also be provided in a retirement home or an assisted living facility. Sometimes a hospice organization has its own residential center.

Hospice has been around for more than 30 years, but it looks very different today than it did 10 years ago. No longer do the majority of hospice patients have a cancer diagnosis. In fact, less that half of all hospice patients have cancer. More than fifty percent of all hospice patients have diseases like dementia, emphysema, heart, and kidney disease. Some patients have no active disease yet still qualify for hospice because they are slowly deteriorating with weight loss and weakness. Everyone who dies and their families can receive benefit from hospice care. Getting into hospice early could help the patient stay in their own home and prevent the caregiver from burning out. Hospice care can also reduce expenses, as Medicare and other insurances will pay for medications, medical supplies and equipment and help with *in home* care.

Why do people refuse such a wonderful benefit? Usually because they have misunderstandings about hospice care or because they are afraid. There is the thought that if the person goes into hospice they will die sooner. This is incorrect. Research shows that people who go into hospice care may actually live longer than those who did not receive hospice care. 26 Some people fear that if they elect to use hospice, then their doctor will no longer offer treatments that will prolong life. This is also incorrect. There is research to show that hospice patients are offered more education and treatment options that those patients who did not elect hospice care. The reality is, that you are free to leave hospice care at any time. Should your doctor offer a new treatment you can sign off hospice and return at a later date. There is no penalty or loss of service days.

When hospice care is added to the care an individual is receiving from a health care provider, there are several important benefits. Hospice has experts who will manage pain and other symptoms. Hospice will help to develop a plan to keep the patient in familiar surroundings in their final months, if that is their wish. This plan will put into place all of the necessary services—counseling services and someone to help with bathing—emergency medications and oxygen in the home before they are needed. A 24-hour-per-day on-call service and a nurse to visit the home whenever needed, even nights and weekends. The hospice staff will visit regularly during the day and will teach you how to take care of your loved one. They will also prepare both patient and caregiver both physically and emotionally for what is coming next. They will help you make decisions and you will feel less alone. Should a situation arise where the patient cannot stay at home, hospice will assist in moving your loved one to an inpatient care setting.

If concerns exist about using hospice care, there is ample opportunity for a trial. First, the service can be tried for a short period of time and it is possible to discontinue if the patient or family decides against it. If the patient is not satisfied with the hospice provider, transfer to another provider is possible. All of this can be done with no penalty or loss of service days.

I am hopeful that the information in this book has made your caregiving experience less stressful and more meaningful. For those who find yourselves advocating for your loved one early in their decline, begin speaking with your family member about their wishes for their own final months. Knowing how they would want medical situations handled will greatly reduce your stress.

It is estimated that as many as 70 percent of adult children have not talked to their parents about their parents' wishes for the final phase of their life. It is never too late. Most people will welcome these conversations. It shows that you care deeply about them, and that you want to honor their wishes. The more information that they share with you, the easier it will be for you to help them make decisions, and later, for you to make the decisions for them.

End Notes

1. Field MJ, Cassel CK, eds. Approaching Death: Improving Care at the End of Life. Washington, DC: National Academy Press; 1997:28-30.
2. Newman A, Yanez D, Harris T, Duxbury A, Enright P and Fried L. Weight change in old age and its association with mortality. *J Am Geriatric Society* 49:1309–1318, 2001.
3. Somes GW et al. Body mass index, weight change and death in older adults. *Am J Epidemiol* 156:132-138, 2002.
4. Murden R, Ainslie NK. Recent weight loss is related to short term mortality in nursing homes. *J General Int Med* 9:648-650, 1994.
5. Koivula I, Steinn M, Makela PH. Risk Factors for pneumonia in the elderly. *Am J Med* 96:313-320, 1994.
6. Loeb M, McGreer A, McArthur M, et al. Risk factors for pneumonia and other lower respiratory tract infections in elderly residents of long term care facilities. *Arch Int Med* 159: 2058-2064, 1999.
7. Marrie TJ, Carriere KC, Jin Y, et al. Mortality during hospitalization for pneumonia in Edmonton Alberta, Canada is associated with physician volume. *Eur Respir J.* 22: 148-155, 2003.
8. Marrie TJ, Wu L, Factors Influencing In-hospital Mortality in Community-Acquired Pneumonia; A Prospective Study of Patients Not Initially Admitted to the ICU. *Chest* 127:1260-1270, 2005.
9. Naughton BJ, Mylotte JM, Tayara A. Outcome of nursing home acquired pneumonia: derivation and application of a practical model to predict 30 day mortality. *JAGS* 48 (10): 1292-1299, 2001.
10. Medina- Walpole AM, McCormick WC. Provider practice patterns in nursing home acquired pneumonia. *JAGS* 46(2):164-169, 1998.
11. Mortensen EM, Kapoor WN, Chang CC, Fine MJ. Assessment of mortality after long-term follow-up of patients with community-acquired pneumonia. *Clin Infect Dis* 37:1617–1624, 2003.
12. Kaplan V, Angus DC, Griffin MF, et al. Hospitalized community acquired pneumonia in the elderly: age and sex related patterns of care and outcome in the United States. *Am J Respiratory Crit Care Med* 165: 766-772, 2002.

13. Waterer GW, Kessler LA, Wunderink RG. Medium-term survival after hospitalization with community-acquired pneumonia. *Am J Respir Crit Care Med* 169: 910–914, 2004.
14. Marik P, Kaplan D. Aspiration pneumonia and dysphagia in the elderly. *Chest* 124: 328-336, 2004.
15. Covinsky KE, Palmer RM, Counsell SR, Pine M, Walter LC, Chren MM Functional status before hospitalization in the acutely ill older adult: validity and clinical importance of retrospective reports. *Journal of the American Geriatric Society* Vol 48,164-169, 2000.
16. Hoyert DL, Aruas E, Smith BL, Murphy SL, Kochanek KD: *National Vital Statistics Reports,* 21 September 2001. (http://www.cdc.gov/nchs/data/nvsr49/nvsr49_08.pdf)
17. Cecil Textbook of Medicine, 21st edition, MB Saunders Co. 2OOO.
18. Keenan SP, Dodek P. Survival as an outcome for ICU patients. *In: Surviving Intensive Care: Update in Intensive Care and Emergency Medicine (Edited by: Angus D, Carlet J).* Berlin: Springer-Verlag 2003, 3-20.
19. Covinsky KE, Palmer RM, Fortinsky RH, Counsell SR, Stewart AL, Kresevic D, et al. Loss of independence in activities of daily living in older adults hospitalized with medical illnesses: increased vulnerability with age. *J Am Geriatric Soc* 51:451-8, 2003.
20. Kaplan V., Angus DC, Griffin MF, Clermont G, Watson RS and Linde-Zwirble WT. Hospitalized community-acquired pneumonia in the elderly age- and sex-related patterns of care and outcome in the United States Clinical Research, Investigation, and Systems Modeling of Acute Illness (CRISMA) Laboratory, Department of Critical Care Medicine, University of Pittsburgh, Pittsburgh; and Health Process Management, Inc.,Doylestown, PA. *Am. J. Respir. Crit. Care Med*, Volume 165, Number 6, March 2002, 766-772.
21. www.alz.org/documents/national/endoflife_brochure.pdf
22. Portenoy RK, Sibirceva U, Smout R, Horn S, Connor S, Blum, Opioid use and survival at the end of life: A survey of a hospice population. *Journal of Pain and Symptom Management.* 32(6): 532-540, 2006.
23. Printz LA. Terminal dehydration; A compassionate treatment. *Archives of Internal Medicine :* 152, 697-700, 1992.

24. McCann R, Hall WJ and Groth-Juncker. Comfort care for terminally ill patients: The appropriate use of nutrition and hydration. *Journal of the American Medical Association*, 272 (16), 1623 – 1626, 1994.
25. Friedman DP: Perspectives on the medical use of drugs of abuse. *J Pain and Symptom Management.* 5:S2-S5, 1990.
26. Connor S, Pyenson B, Fitch K, Spence C, Iwasaki K., Comparing hospice and non-hospice patient survival among patients who die within a three-year window. *Journal of Pain and Symptom Management.*Vol 33, No 3 March 2007.

Quick Order Form
Cost $5.00 each book

Bulk orders are deeply discounted
See:www.GuidetoCaregiving.com

Order by:
FAX : 540-687-6262
Phone : 571-213-3945
Internet: www.GuidetoCaregiving.com
US Postal: TM Brown Publishers
21200 Hibbs Bridge Road
Middleburg, Virginia 20117

Visa, American Ex-
press,Discover,Mastercard

Card No.____________________________exp____
Name_________________________________
Ship to:______________________________
_______________________State____Zip_____

Credit card address for bill (if different from above)

____
_______________________State___Zip______

Shipping:
1-2 books $4
3-10 books $6
11-25 books $9